Chlamydia
the silent disease

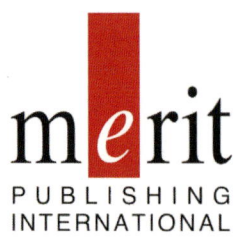

PUBLISHING INTERNATIONAL

European address:
50 Highpoint, Heath Road
Weybridge, Surrey KT13 8TP
England
Tel: (44) (0) 1932 844526
Email: merituk@aol.com
Web: www.meritpublishing.com

North American address:
1095 Jupiter Park Drive,
Suite 7,
Jupiter, FL 33458
Tel: 561 697 1116
Email: meritpi@aol.com

Acknowledgement

The Editors would like to thank Mrs Joan Pleasance for yet further patience and professionalism in helping to prepare the manuscript.

ISBN: 978-1-873413-99-9

©2008 Euromed Communications Ltd. All rights reserved. No part of this publication may be reproduced, stored in a retrieval system or transmitted in any form or by any means, electronic, mechanical, photocopying, recording, or otherwise, without prior permission of the copyright holder.

Co-published in the United States
with Euromed Communications Ltd.

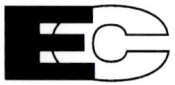

Euromed Communications Ltd
The Old Surgery, Liphook Road, Haslemere,
Surrey GU27 1NL, England
Tel: +44 (0)1428 656665   Fax: +44 (0)1428 656643
email: info@euromed.uk.com

Chlamydia
the silent disease

Edited by
Timothy R Moss
and
Alison J Woodland

Foreword by
Barbara Van Der Pol

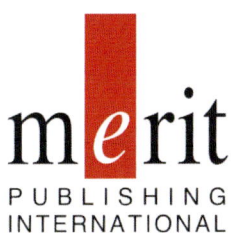

Contents

FOREWORD   VII

Chapter 1   1
Introduction   1
   What is Chlamydia exactly?   1
   How infectious is Chlamydia?   1
   Does catching Chlamydia lead to immunity?   2

Chapter 2   3
Symptoms   3
   What symptoms might it cause?   3

Chapter 3   5
Screening and Diagnosis   5
   Chlamydia Screening Programs?   5
   How do I know if I have Chlamydia?   6

Chapter 4   7
Female complications   7
   What damage can it cause?   7
   Inflammation of the Urethra (Chlamydial Urethral Syndrome)   9
   Inflammation of the Cervix (Cervicitis)   9
   Inflammation of the lining of the Womb (Endometritis)   10
   Pelvic Inflammatory Disease (PID)   11
   Complications of PID   13
   Inflammation of the glands/ducts in the lower Vagina (Bartholinitis)   15

Fitz-Hugh-Curtis Syndrome (FHCS – Peri-hepatitis)	15
Pregnancy and the newborn	17
Reactive arthritis (Reiter's Syndrome)	18

Chapter 5 — 19
Male Complications — 19
What damage can it cause?	19
Inflammation of the Urethra (Urethritis)	19
Inflammation of the Epididymis (Epididymitis)	21
Inflammation of the Prostate (Prostatitis)	22
Inflammation of the Rectum (Proctitis)	22
Reactive arthritis (Reiter's Syndrome)	23

The outlook for men — 24
Why should men be regularly tested?	24

Chapter 6 — 27
Treatment — 27
What will cure this infection?	28

Established drugs — 28
Antibiotics are only half the story — 29
Especially for women — 29
Has my PID been cured? — 31
Especially for men — 31
Conclusions — 32

Chapter 7 — 33
Contact tracing/partner notification — 33

Foreword

Chlamydia trachomatis is a well recognized sexually transmitted infection which, if untreated, has serious consequences. Understanding how to prevent this disease and how to recognize infection is critical for maintaining reproductive health. Unfortunately, this is a disease that is often unnoticeable. As a result of this, infected individuals may not know when to seek treatment and may inadvertently pass this infection on to sexual partners. This book is intended to provide information useful to any reader regarding who is at risk; how to recognize that you may have the disease; how to get tested; consequences of not knowing if you are infected; and, how to cure the infection and stop its spread.

While prevention of infection is the most desirable situation, this "silent" infection can occur in anyone. Both men and women are at risk for chlamydia and need to be aware of how to deal with this disease. It is particularly important for young men and women, who are at the highest risk for contracting this disease, to be informed about the availability of testing and treatment in order to avoid the numerous complications that can occur even from infections that caused no noticeable illness. This Chlamydia handbook is a useful guide for facilitating sexual and reproductive health by providing readers with easy to understand descriptions of this disease and the ways in which it can be dealt with.

Barbara Van Der Pol, PhD, MPH
Director, STD Behavioral Sciences Program
Director, Infectious Diseases Laboratory
Indiana University School of Medicine

Chapter 1

INTRODUCTION

What is Chlamydia exactly?

Chlamydia trachomatis (to give it its full Latin name) is the commonest bacterial sexually transmitted infection affecting millions of people worldwide.

Over the past decade uncomplicated genital Chlamydial infections doubled to over 1,000,000 cases in the USA and continues to rise. It is now the highest ever nationally recorded disease in any year. The picture is similar in the UK where the number of reported cases rose to over 100,000 over the same period.

It most commonly affects sexually active young women aged 16–19 years and men in their early twenties, but clearly all age groups of people who have unprotected sex may be at risk. It is known as the silent disease, as so many people do not know that they have become infected.

Other types of Chlamydia trachomatis cause respiratory (non-sexually transmitted) human infections. This book concentrates solely on Chlamydia trachomatis as a human sexually transmitted infection.

How infectious is Chlamydia?

After just one episode of unprotected sex with an infected person, about 10% will catch Chlamydia.

The reason that this infection is such a problem worldwide, results from its ability to hide inside the cells of the genital tract in both men and women. This means that Chlamydia is passed on in new relationships, with each partner remaining totally unaware.

Does catching Chlamydia lead to immunity?

Sadly, no. You can catch Chlamydia again and again. There is no vaccine, therefore safe sex is the only option.

In women the untreated infection can spread through the womb and along the Fallopian tubes, resulting in Pelvic Inflammatory Disease (PID). This can lead to chronic pelvic pain, infertility and potentially fatal ectopic pregnancy (where the baby develops in the Fallopian tube).

In men, complications are fewer but the infection can spread to the epidydimis (the tubules that carry sperm from the testes) causing pain, inflammation and rarely sterility.

Sometimes, complications of Chlamydial infection can result in a type of arthritis (Reiter's Syndrome) where the joints become inflamed along with the eyes and urethra.

Studies have shown that this bacteria actually enters the cells lining the genital tract, oral and anal membranes and can remain there for years if not treated.

These problems will be discussed in more detail later.

Chapter 2

SYMPTOMS

What symptoms might it cause?

Frequently, none! It is at this point that Chlamydia has the opportunity to cause great damage, with women paying the ultimate price: loss of fertility. This is because 80% of women and 70% of men display no symptoms whatsoever (asymptomatic). Thus life goes on as normal with no-one the wiser that this silent infection is wreaking havoc with their reproductive organs, not to mention the fact that, without the use of condoms, this infection is so easily passed on.

If symptoms do occur, it can take between 1–3 weeks after coming into contact with Chlamydia before they appear or they may be so mild that they remain unnoticed and it is many months later that damage becomes apparent.

If this happens it does not necessarily mean that your partner has been unfaithful. There is a fair chance that he or she developed a Chlamydial infection before your relationship began and had no idea that they were infected.

For the women that do display symptoms the most common are:

An increased vaginal discharge
Pain when passing urine (dysuria)
Lower abdominal pain
Pain during intercourse
Bleeding between periods and/or after sex
If the eyes are affected, (not common) irritation/redness and pain (conjunctivitis)

For the men:

A clear or opaque discharge from the penis
Pain or burning when passing urine (dysuria).
Conjunctivitis if the eyes are infected (not common).

If the rectum is infected there will be little in the way of symptoms but it may cause anal discharge and discomfort. Chlamydial infection of the throat has no symptoms.

Remember, anyone may catch Chlamydia from unprotected vaginal, anal or oral sex or by immediately sharing sex toys without washing them or covering with a new condom each time they are used.

Having Chlamydia can mean you are at more risk of becoming infected with HIV.

You cannot catch Chlamydia from hugging, kissing, sharing baths or towels, from swimming pools, toilet seats or from sharing cups, plates or cutlery, toothbrushes, bedding or clothing.

Chapter 3

SCREENING AND DIAGNOSIS

Chlamydia Screening Programs

The high levels of illness and severe complications of untreated Chlamydial infection have become a major Public Health problem in virtually all nations/countries. There has been a range of screening strategies implemented in the USA and in other countries but each has achieved different success rates.

US Infertility Prevention Project

Based on a demonstration project carried out in the Northwestern region of the US, in 1992 the federal govenment funded the Infertility Prevention Program (IPP). This program provides screening, counseling and treatment for Chlamydia as well as education for providers and clients. Screening through this program is made available at federally and locally sponsored family planning and STD clinics. The findings from this control program have led to the national recommendation that all women under the age of 25 should be tested at least annually.

The program is now expanding to provide testing to people who might not access family planning services in an attempt to further reduce Chlamydia infection rates. New sites for testing include high schools and detention centers.

UK National Chlamydia Screening Programme

During the late 1990s the National Screening Committee in the UK supported a pilot screening program in the Wirral and Portsmouth followed by a roll out of a National Chlamydia Screening Programme

(NCSP) across Britain. This began in ten areas across the UK in 2002. The program then expanded to another 16 areas, with further screening now being provided by Primary Care Trusts. The NCSP offers testing to men and women under the age of 25 years attending a variety of clinical and non-clinical settings. Urine and self-taken vulvo-vaginal swabs are tested.

The NCSP may help control Chlamydial infection but the greatest impact is dependent on diligent attention to 'sexual safety'. It has never been more urgent to consider: new partner equals new condom every time!

Regardless of the screening program, if there has been unprotected sex, ideally a full sexually transmitted infection screen should be carried out. It is important to be aware that it may take several days (or longer) for the infection to become detectable.

How do I know if I have Chlamydia?

Nobody knows without being tested! Diagnosis is dependent on an adequate sample being obtained. If it is a urine sample, it is ideal to have held urine in the bladder for 2–3 hours before it is taken. It is the first 10–20ml of urine that are required not the usual mid-stream sample that is used to test for cystitis.

If a swab is taken in a clinical setting it will usually be taken from the entrance to the cervix (cervical canal). However, many healthcare providers are now collecting vaginal swabs or allowing patients to collect swabs themselves. This avoids the need for a speculum-based pelvic exam in those cases where it would not be performed for other reasons.

No Chlamydia test is perfect but those now available are excellent when requested appropriately and performed accurately.

These tests are based on nucleic acid technology and are much more reliable than earlier test systems.

Chapter 4

FEMALE COMPLICATIONS

What damage can it cause?

Chlamydial infection in women can vary from having absolutely no symptoms whatsoever to a severe illness associated with serious long-term complications, particularly affecting fertility.

Even in females with no symptoms, ongoing damage to the Fallopian tubes may be happening and it is only years later that this comes to light. This usually becomes apparent when there is a failure to fall pregnant.

Chlamydia enters the body through penetrative sex and commonly causes problems in the urethra and cervix and occasionally in the rectum.

The infection can travel up through the womb (uterus) and along the Fallopian tubes and into the pelvis causing pelvic inflammatory disease (PID). It can also then spread throughout the abdomen.

In the Fallopian tubes, inflammation occurs leading to scarring and destruction of the tiny hairs (cilia) lining the tubes. These cilia are vital to carry the fertilized egg along the tube into the womb establishing a pregnancy.

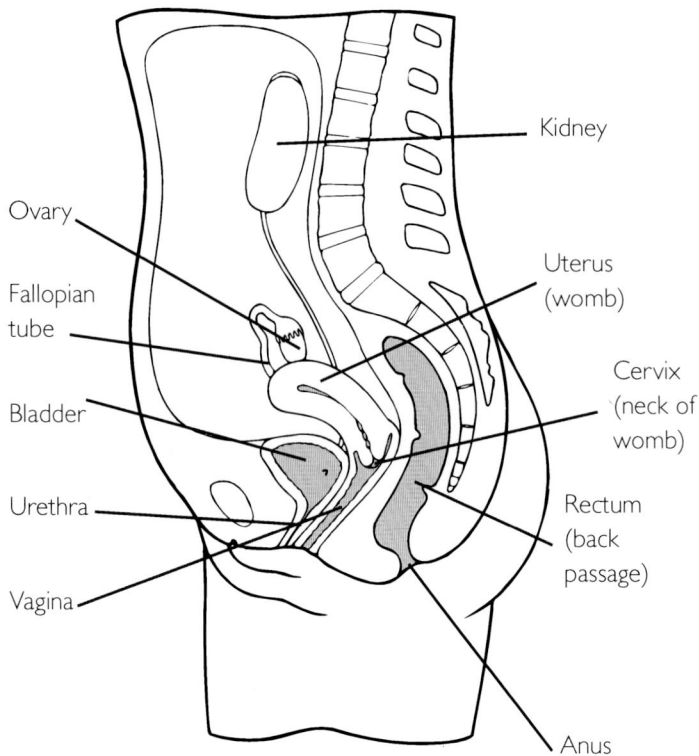

Sometimes this infection can be transferred from the genitals to the eyes by unwashed fingers or occasionally following oral sex.

Anal sex can result in inflammation/pain in the rectum (proctitis). This is less common in women, as is a sore throat (pharyngitis) from oral sex.

If a pregnant woman is infected with Chlamydia this bacteria can be passed to the baby during delivery particularly affecting the eyes (conjunctivitis), and occasionally the lungs (pneumonitis).

Symptoms may appear soon after infection or many months later and just as in adults, untreated, hidden (latent) infection may be reactivated at a later date.

INFLAMMATION OF THE URETHRA (Chlamydial Urethral Syndrome)

The majority of women with Chlamydial infection of this site have no symptoms but occasionally experience a condition called acute urethral syndrome.

There may be a discharge, redness or swelling of the urethral opening (meatus). This syndrome should be considered if symptoms of cystitis go on for more than a week especially if there is no abdominal tenderness.

INFLAMMATION OF THE CERVIX (Cervicitis)

As with all forms of Chlamydial infection, women may not have any symptoms at all. Some however, complain of a discharge. This may be clear or cloudy yellow. There can also be bleeding following sex.

Cervicitis caused by Chlamydia can affect the cervical smear process (screening for pre-cancerous cells in the cervix or "Pap smear") resulting in an inadequate sample.

A negative smear with a comment advising that 'inflammatory changes are present' may indicate a need for Chlamydia testing.

Following the introduction of the new liquid based cervical screening technology a report identifying borderline cell changes may similarly suggest that Chlamydia testing may be appropriate.

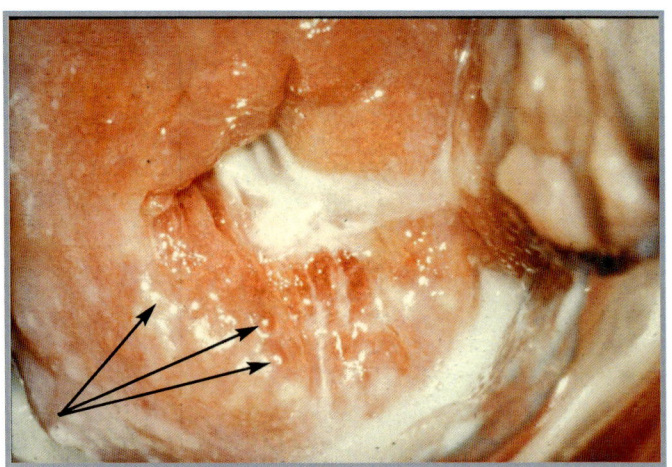

This picture shows the tiny follicles which appear when Chlamydial infection has been present in the neck of the womb for a very long period of time.

INFLAMMATION OF THE LINING OF THE WOMB (Endometritis)

Almost half of the women with Chlamydial cervicitis will also have this condition. Again there may be no signs or it can cause heavy, painful bleeding and bleeding following sex.

An unexpected change in the pattern of periods/menstruation is also suggestive of endometritis.

PELVIC INFLAMMATORY DISEASE (PID)

Pelvic inflammatory disease occurs when the bacteria have travelled from the cervix into the womb and along the Fallopian tubes, causing inflammation (salpingitis) alone or in addition to endometritis.

This can be mild or severe, ongoing or completely silent. Up to 40% of women with Chlamydia will develop PID. There is often infection with other bacteria at the same time (secondary infection).

Teenage girls are most affected by Chlamydia and the risk of developing PID is also greatest in this group. Contraceptive coils increase the risk of Chlamydia causing PID particularly at the first insertion or at subsequent changes. The risk of Chlamydia causing inflammation of the Fallopian tubes (salpingitis) is also increased if a woman decides to terminate a pregnancy or during other gynecological procedures. Testing for Chlamydia before any of these procedures has now reduced these risks.

Recurrences or flare-ups of PID are frequent and can be due to treatment not being completed properly, re-infection from a non-treated partner or a new, infected partner. Re-infection and further episodes of PID cause greater and greater damage.

Other bacteria getting into the genital tract and reaching the already damaged tubes can occur, giving rise to these flare-ups.

The classical symptoms of PID are severe lower abdominal or pelvic pain. There may also be pain on deep sexual penetration, bleeding from the vagina, vaginal discharge and on occasion a high temperature.

Examination by a Doctor can reveal abdominal tenderness and also pain on moving the cervix. However in silent PID there are no symptoms or signs although damage is still occurring in the tubes.

Previous sterilization involving tying of the tubes does not prevent PID.

Diagnosis can be difficult. For a definite diagnosis of severe PID a laparoscopy may be performed but this procedure carries its own additional risks. During laparoscopy an endoscope/'telescope' is inserted through the abdomen and used to directly observe the womb, tubes and ovaries. Often the liver edge is also inspected visually. This procedure is usually performed under a general anesthetic.

The diagnosis of PID, therefore, is made by the Doctor examining/observing/finding signs, taking swabs and evaluating the response to treatment.

If PID is suspected, treatment should be started quickly, especially in adolescents, as even a three-day delay in medication can cause a threefold rise in the risk of infertility.

In sexually active young women and other high-risk groups who display abdominal/womb tenderness or pain on moving the cervix during examination, treatment should be given if no other cause of the illness can be identified.

If a coil is present it may be safer to remove it but only if alternative contraception is available.

Whenever PID is diagnosed other Sexually Transmitted Infections should be tested for (as STIs hunt in packs) – a pregnancy test should be considered in case of tubal (ectopic) pregnancy.

COMPLICATIONS OF PID

As PID worsens abscesses can form on the ovaries and inflammation of the abdominal cavity can develop as well as Fitz-Hugh-Curtis Syndrome (peri-hepatitis) where the liver edge is involved.

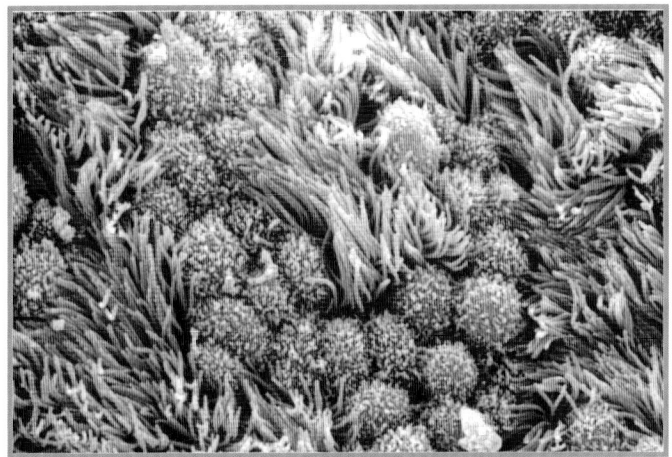

This electron micrograph shows the healthy tiny hairs which form the egg transport system/mechanism. (Magnified 2,600 times)

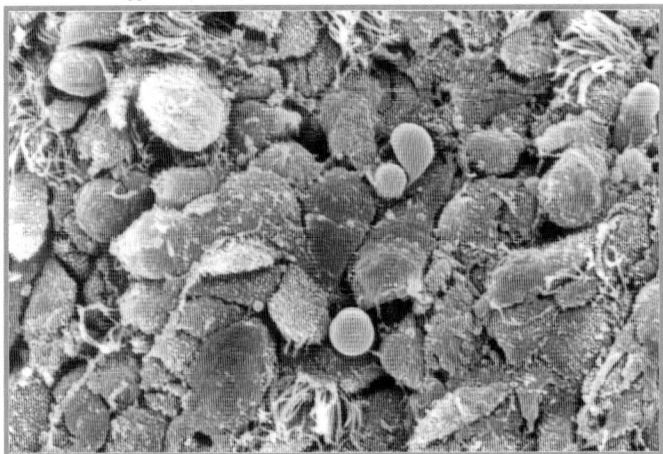

This electron micrograph shows the destruction of this vital 'egg transport mechanism' following infection with Chlamydia. (Magnified 2,600 times)

The long-term complications include ectopic pregnancy, tubal infertility (Fallopian tubes are blocked because of scarring) and the chronic (life-long) pelvic pain that can destroy the quality of women's lives.

By now, the cells lining the Fallopian tubes are sensitive to Chlamydia and the cilia are rapidly destroyed.

For every episode of PID the risk of complications increases greatly.

Ectopic pregnancy is life threatening and causes 1 in 10 of pregnancy related deaths. The risk of an ectopic pregnancy following an episode of PID increases by up to 10 times.

Death from massive bleeding after a ruptured tubal pregnancy is much more common in resource poor countries where emergency healthcare is limited.

Almost half of tubal pregnancies result from Chlamydial infection.

The tubal damage, which occurs as a result of inflammation, scarring and sensitivity, can result in infertility.

About half of all cases of infertility are due to tubal problems of which Chlamydia is the commonest cause. Many give no history of PID.

Chronic pelvic pain occurs in 15% of women with a previous history of PID and, as mentioned above, increase markedly following each episode.

INFLAMMATION OF THE GLANDS/DUCTS IN THE LOWER VAGINA (Bartholinitis)

These ducts (gland openings) are found on each side of the lower vagina. They become blocked by infection, leading to abscess formation. The infection is frequently due to the bacteria that cause gonorrhea, but Bartholinitis can also be due to Chlamydia. Symptoms are typically pain and swelling. On examination a large, tender, swollen abscess on one side of the vaginal entrance will be seen.

FITZ-HUGH-CURTIS SYNDROME (FHCS – Peri-hepatitis)

This term is used to describe the spread of Chlamydia to inflame the tissue covering the liver. Chlamydial infection at this site causes inflammation at the liver edge and the surrounding lining of the abdomen (peritoneum). There is no involvement of the liver itself, just the capsule.

This condition occurs in at least 1 in 5 women with pelvic inflammatory disease.

It results from the spread of Chlamydia from the Fallopian tubes and up through the abdominal lining (peritoneum).

The main symptom is pain around the liver area (under the lowest right rib) with a vaginal discharge and/or pelvic inflammatory disease. Fever, nausea and vomiting can also be symptoms.

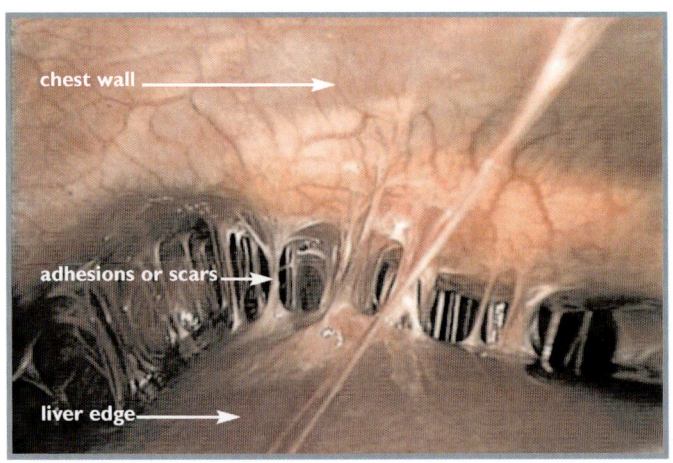

This picture shows the adhesions or scars between the liver edge and chest wall associated with Chlamydia which has spread throughout the abdomen.
This is the so-called Fitz-Hugh-Curtis Syndrome
(Image reprinted with permission from eMedicine.com, 2007.
Available at: http://www.emedicine.com/med/topic797.htm)

The pain can spread to the back and shoulder area and may be made worse by breathing, coughing or movement.

The right upper abdominal pain can present first and be so severe that subsequent PID symptoms go unnoticed. Women with FHCS may adopt a posture leaning to the right.

Diagnosis is usually made by the Doctor's clinical examination and swab tests. A laparoscopy will give a definitive diagnosis where the liver edge and abdominal lining are inflamed and in more advanced cases adhesions (strings of fibrous tissue) between the liver and the abdominal wall will have formed.

PREGNANCY AND THE NEWBORN

After having a baby, inflammation of the lining of the womb (endometritis) is common, occurring in around 30% of women with Chlamydia.

This may lead to tenderness and severe pain in the pelvis, or the condition may be mild or without any symptoms. So if the diagnosis goes unnoticed and therefore untreated, infertility may result (secondary infertility).

Babies of mothers with Chlamydia are at risk of eye problems (conjunctivitis) which develop in up to 50% of cases. Up to 20% of babies may develop Chlamydial pneumonia. The most likely cause is being in contact with infected cervical secretions during birth.

Chlamydial conjunctivitis presents 5-10 days after birth, whereas chest complications (pneumonia) usually occur in babies between 2- 3 weeks old.

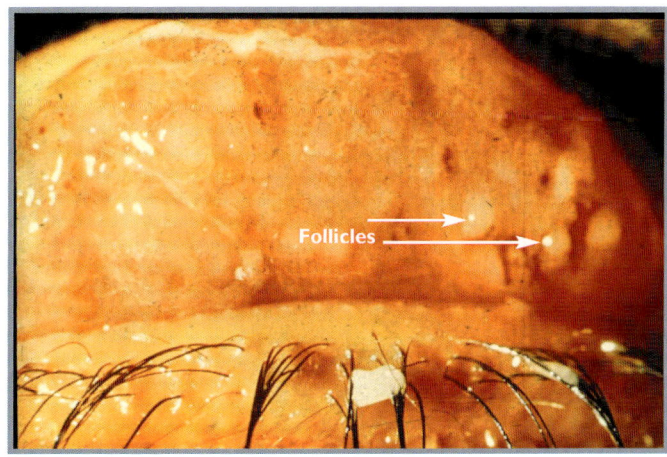

Long-term (chronic) Chlamydial infection of the eyelid with tiny follicles similar to those on the infected cervix (see page 10).

REACTIVE ARTHRITIS
(Reiter's Syndrome)

This condition is diagnosed if a woman has inflammation of the eye (conjunctivitis), inflammation of the joints (arthritis) and inflammation of the urethra (urethritis) all at the same time.

It is much more commonly diagnosed in males than in females (it may not be recognized so easily in women).

The joint inflammation particularly affects the large weight bearing joints and occurs several weeks after infection.

Treatment will be required for the underlying Chlamydial infection along with anti-inflammatory medication, physiotherapy and possibly bed-rest.

Chapter 5

MALE COMPLICATIONS

What damage can it cause?

Around 70% of men display no symptoms when infected with Chlamydia.

The incidence is highest for men between the ages of 20 and 24 years but can affect all sexually active males. A third of the infected population remain blissfully unaware of its presence.

Chlamydia not only infects the urethra. It causes inflammation of the sperm collecting tubules (epididymitis) and may cause inflammation of the prostate (prostatitis). The eyes and the rectum can also be sites of infection.

INFLAMMATION OF THE URETHRA (Urethritis)

Many men show no symptoms at all but for those that do, inflammation of the urethra with or without a discharge, burning when passing urine or irritation of the urethra can be experienced.

Less common symptoms include frequency or urgency in passing urine, including during the night (nocturia) along with swelling of the sperm collecting tubules around the testicle.

Microscopic evidence of urethritis depends upon how many defense (immune) cells can be seen under the microscope.

Looking at a sample under the microscope can tell the difference between a specific infection with gonorrhea in the urethra and a non-specific infection where another organism is present. Hence, microscopy rapidly identifies Non-Specific-Urethritis (NSU). Further laboratory testing will diagnose/identify Chlamydia in half the samples. The other half is often due to other STIs that cannot yet be routinely tested for.

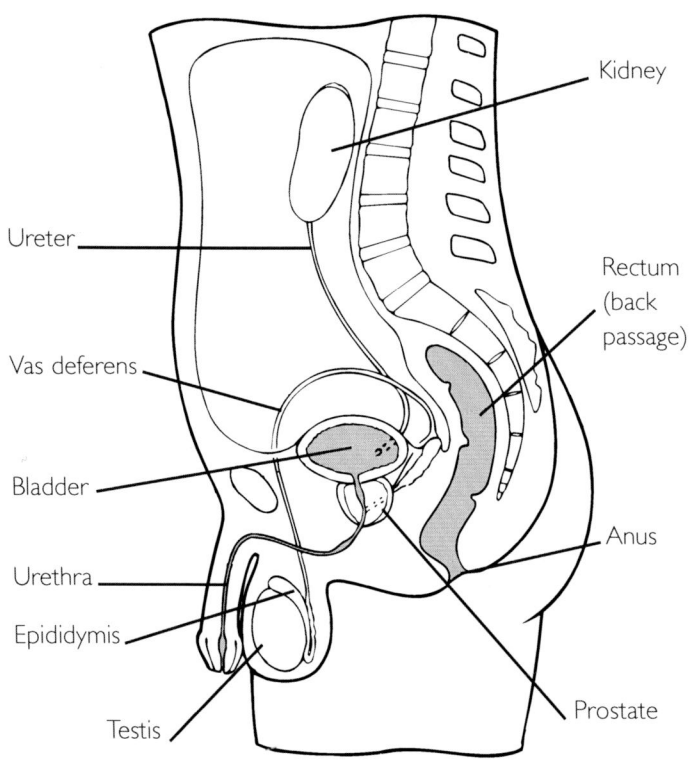

INFLAMMATION OF THE EPIDIDYMIS (Epididymitis)

Chlamydia is a major cause of epididymitis in sexually active men of any age.

Often it's a younger man with urethritis, which may show no symptoms, who goes on to develop a one-sided pain in the scrotum with increasing swelling. However, there are other conditions that give rise to similar symptoms, which can be ruled out by special non-invasive scans.

Chlamydial epididymitis is apparently less destructive to this area unlike the havoc it wreaks in the female reproductive organs, but unlike the loss of fertility caused by Chlamydial pelvic inflammatory disease, the true impact of Chlamydia on male fertility has not yet been fully established.

Although prompt diagnosis and treatment of Chlamydia appears to have a favorable effect on male fertility, a recent report indicates that untreated Chlamydia may damage sperm genetic material (DNA).

This initial research suggests that the fertility of men infected with Chlamydia may be reduced to about one third of that of healthy men. The number of sperm, their quality and swimming ability may also be reduced.

The good news is that when these less fertile men were treated with extended antibiotics the damage to their sperm DNA improved by about a third over a period of 4 months.

INFLAMMATION OF THE PROSTATE (Prostatitis)

This can be either acute (sudden onset) or chronic (gradual onset/long term).

In the acute condition fever, tiredness, frequency of passing urine and pain are the most common symptoms but occasionally acute retention of urine can occur (this is when urine cannot be passed for hours and the bladder becomes over full).

Chronic prostatitis has less severe symptoms. The most common bladder problem includes dribbling of urine after emptying and there may also be a urethral discharge.

A dull, aching pain deep in the lower abdomen, radiating into the area between the testicles and the anus (perineum) is common and can affect the testicles, penis and groin too.

There is no absolute evidence that Chlamydia causes inflammation of the prostate but some men respond extremely well to longer courses of antibiotics. It may be that the association between Chlamydia and prostatitis is part of the male body's reaction to the bacteria. In other words, it is more like an allergic response (sensitivity), rather than a true infection.

INFLAMMATION OF THE RECTUM (Proctitis)

When symptomatic, this condition gives rise to rectal pain, diarrhea, a bloody discharge and the persistent feeling of wanting to go to the toilet (tenesmus). It may be difficult to differentiate this from other bowel conditions.

Many gay men are asymptomatic but are diagnosed during routine testing for sexually transmitted infections.

A diagnosis of Chlamydial proctitis is made from a positive swab/culture taken from the rectum, along with a good response to appropriate treatment.

In gay men in the UK a different type of Chlamydial proctitis has re-emerged caused by Chlamydial 'Lymphogranuloma'(LGV) and can be differentiated on testing as a separate Chlamydial organism.

REACTIVE ARTHRITIS
(Reiter's Syndrome)

This syndrome in the male is defined as inflammation of the joints (arthritis) along with inflammation of the urethra (urethritis) which has been present for more than a month.

A classic presentation of arthritis, urethritis and inflammation of the eye (conjunctivitis) is less common.

It can often be misdiagnosed as one of the other types of arthritis.

This syndrome is a collection of symptoms, which may be easy to diagnose if all three sites (eyes, urethra, and joints) are involved but unfortunately, less than a third of men present like this. However, if a patient can give a good sexual history it will help enormously in diagnosing this condition.

Urethritis is an early symptom, showing within 2–4 weeks after sex. Prostatitis may also be present. Half of all cases will have eye complications. The swollen painful joints of arthritis are usually the last feature to appear.

Any joint may be affected but the favored sites are the ankles, knees and toes with the fingers and wrists becoming involved as the disease progresses. Fifty per cent of patients will have inflammation affecting the lower back (sacro-iliac joints). In some, the inflammation can affect tendons and ligaments too, particularly the Achilles tendon (back of heel) and the sole of the foot (plantar fascia).

Around half of men with Reiter's syndrome will develop painless shallow ulcers on the lips, roof of the mouth and tongue and a rash on the penis (circinate balanitis).

Unusual complications are inflammation of the membrane covering the heart (myocarditis) and occasionally tingling or numbness in the hands and feet (peripheral neuropathy). Joint fluid may reveal an increased white cell count (an increase in immune or defense cells in the blood).

THE OUTLOOK FOR MEN

Why should men be regularly tested?

Because men are notoriously unreliable when it comes to using condoms!

This frequently silent disease presents a real and increasing danger to the sexual health of men, both physically and psychologically. Because it often shows no symptoms, Chlamydia commonly goes undiagnosed. Improved, less invasive tests will hopefully make them much more acceptable.

This will facilitate screening which should reveal more of this hidden infection in both males and females and thereby reduce the infection rate and the number of complications it causes.

Women have historically been seen as the ideal population to screen since they willingly go to Family Planning, Antenatal and Well Women Clinics. These are ideal locations for sexually active women to be screened effectively.

With men, however, the situation is very different. Men are said to be 80 times more likely to take their car to be checked than visit their Doctor. At present there is no formal focus on healthcare for young men.

This lack of healthcare provision encourages men to leave the responsibility for care and control of sexually transmitted infections to women, along with contraception and termination of pregnancy.

Some Genito-Urinary (GU) clinics have provided 'couples' clinics for many years in order to encourage and develop shared sexual responsibility. They have been proven to be very effective and popular but there are not enough clinics across the country to deal with the number of people needing STI care or indeed this important approach to STI care.

Chapter 6

TREATMENT

What will cure this infection?

The obvious aim of course is to clear the body of Chlamydial infection and ensure a cure. We know, however, many people infected with Chlamydia have no symptoms and their partners may or may not be infected. The serious nature of complications highlights the need for safe, effective Chlamydial treatment with minimal side effects.

Research studies tell us which type or 'family' of antibiotics will work against Chlamydia and which will not.

Some antibiotics only partially treat the infection. This makes us feel better, the symptoms improve but the infection, instead of clearing, is only masked and what is left is hidden (latent infection).

Infections resistant to antibiotics are well known. To reduce the opportunity for Chlamydia to become resistant to antibiotics, all medication must be taken as prescribed, to the letter.

ESTABLISHED DRUGS

Only two families of antibiotics are widely used in treating Chlamydia effectively. These are the Tetracyclines and Macrolides. A third family – the Quinolones, has also been used.

Tetracyclines have been shown to clear Chlamydia from the male urethra within 7, 14 or 21 days therapy, with failure rates of around 3%.

In women with Chlamydial cervical infection, tetracycline is effective if taken carefully along with avoidance of sex during treatment.

Single doses are not effective with this class of antibiotic.

Doxycycline and minocycline belong to the Tetracycline family.

Erythromycin and azithromycin belong to the Macrolide family.

Ofloxacin belongs to the Quinolone family.

Doxycycline 100mg taken twice a day for seven days is a standard therapy with which all new antibiotic regimens have been compared. It should be taken after food to decrease stomach upsets. Occasionally a sensitivity to sunlight may cause skin redness and discomfort whilst taking the medication. Indigestion remedies should not be taken with tetracyclines as this interferes with the absorption of the antibiotic. This family of antibiotics is not recommended for use in pregnancy.

Erythromycin is the alternative here. It is safe in pregnancy but can cause vomiting, diarrhea and stomach cramps. To be effective it has to be taken twice a day for two weeks. Erythromycin has important drug interactions, for example, with some modern anti allergy medication.

Azithromycin is well established as a single dose therapy but only for early, uncomplicated infection. It may be more useful for people with chaotic life styles which make it difficult for them to adhere to treatment regimens or to attend follow up clinics.

Ofloxacin is an alternative antibiotic that can be used successfully in the treatment of Chlamydial infection. Occasionally adverse reactions such as dizziness and feeling a bit low have been reported. There is a risk of drug interaction with non-steroidal anti-inflammatory drugs such as brufen and diclofenac causing these side effects.

Some antibiotics, e.g. from the penicillin family, that are commonly used for urinary tract infections (cystitis) are not effective in treating Chlamydial infections. Be aware, even the best Chlamydial treatment has a failure rate and re-treatment may be required. This emphasizes the importance of attending for a test of cure.

ANTIBIOTICS ARE ONLY HALF THE STORY

In sexual infections, the social and sexual behavior of infected persons with Chlamydia can have a significant influence on the success of the therapy.

Patients and partners should understand the infection, the treatment prescribed and how to take it – and the need for contact tracing along with abstinence from sex during treatment and the benefits of completing treatment.

ESPECIALLY FOR WOMEN

When Chlamydia occurs together with other sexual infections a different antibiotic approach for each individual infection may be recommended.

Remember, antibiotic treatment for Chlamydia may interact with the contraceptive pill and patch and there must be no sexual activity until both you and your partner/partners have completed treatment.

In pregnancy effective treatment is essential to avoid the baby becoming infected at the time of birth. When clinical problems occur in the baby the site most commonly affected is the eye. Oral erythromycin suspension is the preferred antibiotic for treating infants.

Chloramphenicol eye ointment is often routinely sold in Pharmacies or prescribed by Doctors for conjunctivitis. It is not an effective treatment in either babies or adults with Chlamydial conjunctivitis.

Pelvic inflammatory disease (PID) can present itself in many different ways, the most important being the mild or silent type.

Any suspicion of undiagnosed acute or chronic pelvic pain in a patient should be treated.

There is evidence to suggest that delay in treatment can increase the risk of damage to the Fallopian tubes leading to infertility.

It is important that all therapy for PID should cover three probable infections – Chlamydia, gonorrhea and anaerobic infection. Anaerobic refers to organisms which thrive in an environment with little oxygen present. They are thought to add to the process of PID as secondary, subsequent or 'opportunistic' infectious agents, known as pathogens.

More serious cases should receive the antibiotics intravenously (directly into a vein) to obtain the best outcome. These should continue for 24 hours after a sustained improvement, before tablets are introduced.

All sexual partners should be given appropriate antibiotics – and there must be no sexual contact until the course of treatment is completed.

HAS MY PID BEEN CURED?

Test of cure is usually regarded as a clinical resolution (when symptoms settle). We would argue that the only long term test of cure is conception and maintained pregnancy in a previously treated woman.

A women who is infertile after successfully treated PID may be in that situation because she has gone on to have further, undiagnosed infection with Chlamydia in her pelvis.

With early diagnosis, specialist care and full treatment of both patient and partner, the future chances of successful pregnancy are usually favorable.

ESPECIALLY FOR MEN

Chlamydia can spread to the male sperm collection system: the epidydimes, causing epidydimitis.

The rules remain the same; treat with an antibiotic that covers Chlamydia, gonorrhea and other urogenital organisms e.g. mycoplasmas, ureaplasmas.

The prostate can become involved, causing prostatitis. There is controversy as to whether Chlamydia is actually the cause. Nevertheless, long courses of antibiotics have improved symptoms dramatically in some cases.

Reiter's Syndrome is also known as Sexually Acquired Reactive Arthritis – (SARA).

Prompt treatment of Chlamydial infection may reduce the risk of developing this allergic type reaction, which causes inflammation of the large joints and urethra.

CONCLUSIONS

- There are only a few antibiotic groups that are active against Chlamydia and some are suspected of only containing the infection rather than clearing it.
- The complex nature and long life of this bacteria require high levels of antibiotics over a sustained period of time.
- Successful treatment also depends on the patients' understanding of and compliance in taking an effective antibiotic as prescribed.
- Sexual partners need to be treated also and no sex during treatment is essential.
- The commonest causes of treatment failure are forgetting to take the antibiotics as prescribed and sex during therapy.

Chapter 7

CONTACT TRACING/PARTNER NOTIFICATION

What does this involve?

Whatever the terminology, this is a most important part of care, not least to prevent a newly diagnosed untreated person becoming re-infected.

The objectives are to identify and treat current and recent partners, particularly those who show no symptoms, to reduce re-infection, to reduce the spread of infection within the community and prevent the complications and misery associated with this disease.

Contact tracing begins when a positive Chlamydial diagnosis is given. A discussion with a Health Adviser covers how Chlamydia is spread and the risk to partners who may be showing no symptoms at all.

It should be made very clear that there is a long latent (silent) period associated with Chlamydia in some people.

The Chlamydia test cannot tell how long the infection has been there, so the possibility of re-infection of the patient and sexual partners must be understood if current and future partners are to avoid the disease.

Women, particularly those with Chlamydial pelvic inflammatory disease (PID), should be informed of the risk of ectopic pregnancy.

They should be given advice on getting care quickly if complications develop such as one-sided, deep pelvic pain as well as a delayed period.

The future risk of infertility, particularly if re-infection with Chlamydia occurs, should be discussed.

Women are often greatly distressed to learn of a risk to their future fertility. It is essential to reassure them that early diagnosis and prompt treatment of both themselves and their partner/partners usually prevents complications.

All patients should be advised not to have sex until they and their partner have finished their course of antibiotics and a test of cure performed, if appropriate. Advice on safe sex and the use of condoms should be given.

Patients are encouraged and empowered to cooperate with contact tracing/partner notification but participation remains voluntary in this country. In some countries this is mandatory.

Details of any sexual contacts in the previous three to six months will be requested.

If there have been no partners in this time then the very last partner should be determined however long ago.

The most common method used in partner notification is the issue of contact slips. This relies entirely on the willingness of the patient to pass on a slip to each of their sexual contacts.

The slips contain the date, diagnosis (written in Department of Health code) the hospital of origin and the reference number of the patient – thus maintaining confidentiality.

If the patient is not likely to see the contact again or wishes to remain anonymous, the Health Adviser will contact the sexual partner either by telephone or letter. Very occasionally a home visit is made.

There is also the option of the patient telling their contacts/partners themselves but within an agreed timeframe. If the partner has not attended the clinic for screening by this agreed time the Health Adviser will initiate contact.

For couples in long-term relationships, the opportunity for joint consultation should be provided whenever requested.

This not only facilitates prompt and effective treatment but also protects and even enhances the relationship.

With new technology, other methods of advising contacts to attend clinic are coming on-stream for example: texting/e-mailing or providing a home test kit for patients' partners.

In Europe, only EEC 'Kite Marked' test kits should be used.

As partner notification is discussed as soon as a positive diagnosis is made, a patient can be reassured that his or her identity, or diagnosis will not be disclosed. Remember; confidentiality is guaranteed.

Partner notification remains an essential part of the control of Chlamydia. Its purpose is to protect you, your partner, your relationship and your future, as well as to protect the public against this insidious and potentially devastating disease.